Organic

Perfume Made Easy

55 DIY Natural Homemade Perfume Recipes For
Beautiful And Aromatic Fragrances

Ronnie Alexander

ISBN-13: 978-1505376890

DEDICATION

To Jenny, how much better the world would be if everyone had a sister like you.

TABLE OF CONTENTS

INTRODUCTION

The art of perfume making is pretty easy - anyone can become a master at it. Basically, it is the correct combination of ingredients that even gets better with time. All you need are the supplies, a little imagination and the rest is fun.

It is also an activity that you can enjoy with your kids, a delightful way to spend the evening and achieve your desired fragrance with ease.

Advantages Of Homemade Perfume

These days, an increasing number of people would rather make their own perfume than buy one. Perfume making is easy, fun and extremely economical. Trying various mixes with friends and family is really great fun.

Since it is organic and natural, you are free from any harmful chemical ingredients contained in store-bought products.

The major ingredient (essential oils) is readily available and this wide range of essential oils provides health and holistic benefits to its numerous users.

Generally, the major reason perfumes are worn is the feminine appeal it gives to women. Now, with homemade perfumes, women now have the opportunity of making their own distinct and natural fragrance just the way they like it.

Of course, it is cheaper for them too.

Homemade perfume can be given as a gift and the recipient will definitely appreciate it since it was specially made for him or her.

It is a profitable venture that can provide you with extra source of revenue. For less than 300 dollars, for instance, you can make about 100 bottles of your desired perfume. If you sold a bottle for 10 dollars, you will be making thrice your total investment and providing organic and natural quality product as well.

Essential Oils

Perfume is made up of three major ingredients: essential oils, water and pure grain alcohol. Essential oils are the most crucial ingredient needed for perfume making. Since they are concentrated oils distilled from plants, a great variety of them are available.

Only a few drops are needed for any recipe so it is best to carefully follow the directions when making your perfume. You can always add extra drops if you want a stronger smell. It is impossible to remove the drops once you have made an extremely strong- scented perfume!

Some oils may cause skin irritation. Therefore, be sure to check the specific oil profiles for your chosen recipes. Although there are some essential oils that are safe for pregnant women, it is safer to avoid them all.

Essential oils vary in prices so avoid buying cheap ones or shopping at a store that sell all at the same price. This indicates that the oils may be synthetic.

Do not buy oils stored in plastic bottles as the plastic may contaminate the oils. Do not buy those stored in clear glass bottles either as they tend to make the oil spoil faster. Buy essential oils stored in dark bottles only.

It is also advisable not to smell too many essential oils at once as you nose may become overworked, making it unable to distinguish one scent from another.

If however, you do find that you nose is overworked, a simple way to address the problem is to hold a fresh coffee beans a few inches from your nose and inhale a number of times. Your nose will get back to business in no time.

Citrus oils like Bergamot, Lime, Orange, Grapefruit, Petitgrain, Neroli and Lemon can be photosensitive so they shouldn't be worn in the sun.

Perfumes smell different on different individuals and skin types. As a result, do not be disappointed if you do not like them all. Simply have fun experimenting with the recipes.

<u>Getting Undiluted Essential Oils</u>

Getting pure, quality essential oils is vital to the quality of the perfume because it will affect the fragrance. Compared to essential oil, the therapeutic properties of synthetic oils are of lesser quality. With pure essential oil, you can be sure of a long- lasting quality fragrance.

How to determine the purity of an essential oil

Hold the bottle of essential oil about 5 inches away and you should still be able to get a good smell if it is pure and undiluted. You do not need to put your nose right up to the bottle to get a good whiff.

Another way is to place a drop of it on a piece of paper. Undiluted essential oil will not leave a stain behind.

Perfume Notes & Scents

The categorization of essential oil is what is referred to as notes in perfume making. Notes are simply perfume scents. They are divided into three layers: top, middle and base notes.

A successful perfume must have all three notes combined. Different essential oil can be mixed and matched to get your desired scent. The fragrance must be appealing and long lasting.

Top notes are the immediate scents detected once the blended perfume is worn. They are usually light, smell fresh but evaporate quickly. They include lemon, peppermint, orange, neroli, lemongrass, bergamot and chamomile.

Middle notes become perceivable once the top notes vanish. It helps to conceal any unpleasant fragrance from the base note. It is the heart of the perfume and lasts for several minutes. They include geranium, lavender, ylang ylang, rosewood, jasmine and rose.

Base notes become perceivable after about 20 minutes of wearing it. They serve as a fixative to the top and middle notes to make their aroma last longer. They are usually rich and heavy. Examples of common ones are cinnamon, vanilla, patchouli, sandalwood, cedarwood and clove.

Types Of Scents

The primary reason people make their own perfume is to achieve a particular scent or fragrance. However, many of them are unsure of how to combine the right oils to achieve that specific fragrance.

For example, your husband may like colognes with woodsy fragrance. If you were to buy it in a store, it is easy because it will come with a name. When making yours however, you need a prior knowledge of the essential oils that can be used to achieve this fragrance.

The categorization below will be of help to you:

Floral scent: The main components of floral scents consist of flowers. The scent can be fresh and sweet. It is often used by women. Examples are geranium, jasmine, rose, ylang ylang or neroli essential oils.

Herbal scents: chamomile, rosemary, angelica, basil, lavender, peppermint or clary sage.

Earthy scents: patchouli or vetiver.

Spicy scents: these scents are heavier and more sensual. They include black pepper, cinnamon, cardamom, ginger, clove, juniper, nutmeg, or coriander.

Fruity scents: Fruity component is pronounced in these scents. They are usually combined with floral aromas. They include lime, bergamot, lemon, grapefruit, orange, mandarin or lemongrass.

Woodsy scents loved by men: cypress, cedarwood, pine or sandalwood.

Benefits Of Perfume Ingredients

It is important to know the benefits of the major ingredient to be used for your perfume, their different scent properties and how they all work together to give you the scent that you desire.

Perfumes provide many health benefits to the body. Having this vital information will help you to know the dual perfume your perfume can be put to use.

Vodka serves as perfect carrier oil. It is odorless, enhances the fragrance of the perfume and sustains its durability.

Oils from the skins of citrus fruits make excellent top note for perfume. They provide moderately invigorating scent that can be used for men's cologne and women's perfume as well. Oils that are suitable for men's colognes include cypress, lemongrass and verbena.

Jojoba oil is great choice for base oil. It is waxy, non-greasy, easily absorbable oil made from jojoba seeds. It has an extensive shelf-life as well.

Ylang ylang oil is commonly used for its many properties such as helping to relax the muscles, calming nerves and arousing sexual desire. The most erotic scent ever, it is a great aphrodisiac.

Geranium oil emits a rosy and delicate fragrance and is usually used to reduce fatigue, treat anxiety and stress. Similar in properties to rose essential oil, it is a cheaper alternative and provides harmony and balance

Patchouli oil is a warm fragrance that is earthy as well. It is a wonderful choice for a women's perfume or even a man's cologne. Since it does not evaporate quickly, it is generally used as a fixative. It will also prolong the scent in your perfume.

For aromatherapy purposes:

- Sandalwood and Grapefruit help to fight fear.
- Orange and Ylang ylang help with anger.
- Jasmine and Lavender help in relieving anxiety and aid sleep. Lavender is called the universal oil. It is great for many things, including burns and skin problems.
- Cypress and Rosemary help to build confidence.
- Rosemary works for fatigue as well.
- Frankincense, bergamot and Rose help to deal with grief and depression.
- Peppermint is good for boosting memory power. Peppermint also works well for headaches and migraines relief as well as clearing the mind. It's also ideal for digestion comfort.
- Lemon is soothing and calming on the mind and spirit and helps to lift the spirits.
- Helichrysum and Marjoram are good in helping to fight panic.

Helpful Tips For Perfume Making

- Test essential oils on your skin to be sure you do not react to them.
- The higher the number of essential oil drops that are used, the stronger the perfume.
- Essential oils are only for external use. Keep out of children's reach and never use on cats and birds.
- Do not substitute tap water for distilled water.
- Vodka used must be 100 proof.
- If you desire a little color in your perfume, use only natural vegetable food dye.
- Buy essential oils in bulk. it is cheaper

- Use empty and clean Chapstick tube as storage for solid perfume. It is easy to apply.
- Apply solid perfume moderately on business cards. This smells great!
- Store perfume in a dark bottle or glass container to make it last longer.
- For each essential oil applied, use a separate pipette otherwise wash it in alcohol after each use. This helps to keeps your perfume from being marred or contaminated.
- Do not forget that the longer a perfume sits, the stronger the scent and the more it will last.
- For your perfume to blend well and settle, it may take between 1-3 months so shake the bottle every day.
- If you would like to have a higher incense fragrance in your perfume, add 2-3 drops of Ambrette Seed, Cedar Moss, Copal, Tonka Bean or Benzoin resin.
- They act as fixatives and can therefore offer a stronger and long-lasting perfume. However, use them moderately because they have strong effects.
- Try experimenting and you will come up with some luxurious scents.

BOTANICAL PERFUMES

Exotic Perfume Blend

Ingredients

2 drops palmarosa essential oil

3 drops bergamot essential oil

4 drops sandalwood essential oil

3 drops rose absolute essential oil

½ fluid ounce vodka or any high-proof grain alcohol

Directions

Mix the alcohol and essential oils in a glass bottle. Let it sit for 2 to 6 weeks. Shake to mix occasionally.

Siren Song Perfume

Ingredients

6 tablespoons vodka

9 drops bergamot oil

7 drops sandalwood oil

14 drops rose oil

2 tablespoons carrier oil, preferably jojoba or grapeseed

2 ½ tablespoons distilled or spring water

Directions

1. Place the carrier oil into a curing bottle.

2. Add the essential oils.

3. Add the vodka, place lid on bottle and shake vigorously for some minutes.

4. Let the bottle sit for 2 to 6 weeks. Check the scent regularly.

5. Once you are pleased with it, add the water to the blend. Shake for 1 minute.

6. Get a funnel; place a coffee filter into it and then transfer contents from the curing bottle to a storing bottle.

7. Label and wear.

Fiery Passions Perfume

This perfume has a sensual and exotic aroma that you can't help but love.

Ingredients

3 drops Neroli essential oil

2 drops ylang ylang essential oil

3 drops passionflower essential oil

1/2 pt (300ml) 70 % vodka

Directions

1. Pour the vodka into a dark bottle.

2. Add other ingredients and mix thoroughly.

3. Let the mixture settle for 1 week in a cool and dry area.

4. Dab on pulse points and enjoy your fiery passion perfume.

Rich Floral Perfume Blend

<u>Ingredients</u>

6 drops bergamot essential oil

2 drops jasmine essential oil

2 drops rose absolute essential oil

3 drops sandalwood essential oil

5 drops Vanilla Essentials

½ ounce of sweet almond oil

<u>Directions</u>

Combine all oils. Let it sit for 3- 7days, mixing occasionally.

Victorian Verbena Lavender Scent

<u>Ingredients</u>

1 cup vodka

1½ teaspoons verbena oil

20 drops lavender oil

20 drops bergamot oil

<u>Directions</u>

1. Pour the vodka into a dark bottle.

2. Add other ingredients and mix thoroughly.

3. Let the mixture settle for 1 week in a cool and dry area.

4. Dab on pulse points and enjoy your Victorian scent.

Dew Of Rain Perfume

Pure and refreshing, this perfume is irresistible.

Ingredients

2- 3 cup distilled water

5 -6 drops of sandalwood oil

9 -10 drops bergamot oil

3- 4 tablespoon vodka

Directions

1. Mix the vodka and the essential oils together in a bottle, shaking thoroughly.

2. Let it stay for 3 weeks then add distilled water.

3. Set it aside for 1 week, shaking at least once a day.

4. Store in a cool and dark place.

5. for long-lasting fragrance, dab on pulse points.

Musky floral Perfume Blend

This perfume blend can be used on its own or use as a musk oil alternative to add to other blends.

Ingredients

7 drops myrrh essential oil

9 drops patchouli essential oil

7 drops cedarwood essential oil

9 drops frankincense essential oil

10 drops Vanilla Essentials

1 fluid ounce of carrier oil

Directions

Combine all oils. Let it sit for 3- 7days, mixing occasionally.

Fruitwood Perfume

Fruitwood perfume is a, citrusy scent. The verbena and lemongrass adds a woodsy fragrance to it.

Ingredients

5 tsp vodka

1/2 tsp distilled water

10 drops lemongrass essential oil

10 drops verbena essential oil

10 drops grapefruit oil

15 drops lemon essential oil

3 drops cedarwood oil

5 drops neroli oil

2 drops benzoin oil

Directions

1. Pour the vodka into a dark bottle.

2. Add other ingredients and mix thoroughly.

3. Let the mixture settle for 2-3 weeks in a cool and dry area, shaking and inverting bottle occasionally to blend the scent.

4. Dab on pulse points and enjoy your Victorian scent.

Sweet & Fresh Perfume Blend

Ingredients

2 drops peppermint essential oil

10 drops Vanilla Essentials

9 drops lavender essential oil

½ ounce of carrier oil such as sweet almond oil or grapeseed

Directions

1. Combine all oils. Let it sit for 3- 7days, mixing occasionally.

Midnight Garden

Ingredients

2 tablespoons jojoba oil

15 drops clove oil

6 drops cedarwood oil

9 drops lavender oil

2 1/2 tablespoons spring or distilled water

6 tablespoons vodka

Directions

1. Place the carrier oil into a curing bottle.

2. Add the essential oils.

3. Add the vodka, place lid on bottle and shake vigorously for some minutes.

4. Let the bottle sit for 2 to 6 weeks. Check the scent regularly.

5. Once you are pleased with it, add the water to the blend. Shake for 1 minute.

6. Get a funnel; place a coffee filter into it and then transfer contents from the curing bottle to a storing bottle.

7. Label and wear.

Sweet Floral Perfume Blend

<u>Ingredients</u>

2 drops sweet orange essential oil

2 drops patchouli essential oil

3 drops ylang ylang essential oil

½ ounce vodka or any high-proof grain alcohol

<u>Directions</u>

Mix the alcohol and essential oils in a glass bottle. Let it sit for 2 to 6 weeks. Shake to mix occasionally.

Surprise Perfume

This amazing fragrance will certainly inspire admiration, awe and wonder.

<u>Ingredients</u>

10 drops rosemary essential oil

10 drops cypress essential oil

2 cups distilled water

5 drops St. John's wort

3 tablespoons vodka

<u>Directions</u>

1. Mix together all ingredients in a dark color bottle, shake well.

2. Let it settle for 12-18 hours. Store it in a cool & dry area.

3. Dab on pulse points.

Brighter Day

Ingredients

6 tablespoons vodka

2 tablespoons sweet almond or jojoba carrier oil

14 drops lemongrass oil

7 drops pine oil

9 drops orange oil

2 1/2 tablespoons distilled water

Directions

1. Place the carrier oil into a curing bottle.

2. Add the essential oils.

3. Add the vodka, place lid on bottle and shake vigorously for some minutes.

4. Let the bottle sit for 2 to 6 weeks. Check the scent regularly.

5. Once you are pleased with it, add the water to the blend. Shake for 1 minute.

6. Get a funnel; place a coffee filter into it and then transfer contents from the curing bottle to a storing bottle.

7. Label and wear.

Love Tonic Perfume

Increase your love feelings of love with this pleasant aphrodisiac.

Ingredients

15 drops bergamot essential oil

2 drops vanilla essential oil

3 drops sandalwood essential oil

3 drops cedar-wood essential oil

300ml 70% vodka or alcohol

Directions

1. Pour the vodka or any other kind of alcohol into a jar or bottle.

2. Add the oils, shaking well to mix.

3. Set aside for 1 week before using.

Enchanted Perfume

Truly enchanting, this easy-to-make perfume is also magical!

Ingredients

10 drops sandalwood essential oil

3 tablespoons vodka

2 cups distilled water

10 drops peony essential oil

5 drops everlasting essential oil

Directions

1. Mix together all ingredients in a dark color bottle, shake well.

2. Let it settle for 12-18 hours.

3. Store in a cool & dry area.

4. For a long-lasting fragrance, dab on pulse points.

Jasmine Perfume

Ingredients

2 drops Sandalwood

1 drop Jasmine

1 drop Ylang Ylang

½ to 1 tsp Massage oil

Directions

Blend oils. Apply to pulse points

Nice Night Perfume

Apply to the body, pillow & sheets before bed time to calm the nerves and strengthen the body.

Ingredients

4 drops Sandalwood essential oil

3 drops Frankincense essential oil

4 drops Musk essential oil

2 teaspoons Jojoba oil

Directions

1. Pour all the ingredients into a dark-colored bottle. Shake vigorously to mix.

2. Let it stand for 12-18 hours before using.

3. Keep in a cool, dry place.

Shinning Stars Perfume

Ingredients

2 cups distilled water

5 drops Lavender essential oil

10 drops Chamomile essential oil

10 drops Valerian essential oil

3 tablespoons Vodka

Extra fine body glitter, optional

Directions

1. Pour all the ingredients into a dark-colored bottle. Shake vigorously to mix.

2. Let it stand for 12-18 hours before using.

3. Keep in a cool, dry place

4. Add some extra fine body glitter to oil mixture for added effect.

Raindrops Perfume

<u>Ingredients</u>

10 drops cassis essential oil

5 drops sandalwood essential oil

10 drops bergamot essential oil

3 tablespoons vodka

2 cups distilled water

<u>Directions</u>

1. Pour all the ingredients into a dark-colored bottle. Shake vigorously to mix.

2. Let it stand for 12-18 hours before using.

3. Keep in a cool, dry place.

Forestry Perfume

This blend smells great! It is uplifting and comforting as well.

<u>Ingredients</u>

1 tsp organic Jojoba Oil

4 drops Spruce essential oil

2 drops Cedarwood essential oil

2 drops Fir Needle essential oil

1 drop Bergamot essential oil

1 drop Vetiver essential oil

1. Drip all the essential oils into a glass bottle.

2. Roll the bottle between palms to mix the oils evenly

3. Add Jojoba oil and roll again.

4. If you want a stronger perfume, add more essential oils

Summer Sweet Perfume

This relaxing and warm blend is extremely valuable during the dark winter months.

Ingredients

10 drops Lavender essential oil

1 drop Cedarwood essential oil

5 drops Chamomile essential oil

1 drop Geranium essential oil

4 drops Cardamom essential oil

1 tsp organic Jojoba Oil

Directions

1. Drip all the essential oils into a glass bottle.

2. Roll the bottle between palms to mix the oils evenly

3. Add Jojoba oil and roll again.

4. If you want a stronger perfume, add more essential oils

Rejuvenating Perfume

In three words: Rejuvenating, refreshing and stimulating!

<u>Ingredients</u>

5 drops Juniper Berry essential oil

13 drops Peppermint essential oil

5 drops Lemon essential oil

13 drops Rosemary essential oil

5 drops Sage essential oil

1 tsp Jojoba Oil

<u>Directions</u>

1. Drip all the essential oils into a glass bottle.

2. Roll the bottle between palms to mix the oils evenly

3. Add Jojoba oil and roll again.

4. If you want a stronger perfume, add more essential oils

SOLID PERFUMES

Lemon & Lavender Solid Perfume

Ingredients

3g Beeswax

12g Sweet Almond Oil

5 drop Rosemary essential oil

15 drops lavender essential oil

3 drops lemongrass essential oil

Directions

1. In a small saucepan, melt together the beeswax and sweet almond oil over low heat.

2. Remove from heat and set aside to cool for 1minute.

3. Add the essential oils. Swirl to combine.

4. Pour gently into small 1/4 oz tins. Recipe should fill 2 tins.

Vanilla & Lavender Solid Perfume

<u>Ingredients</u>

30 drops lavender essential oil

4 tbsp sweet almond oil

4 tbsp beeswax

25 drops vanilla oil

1 tsp of raw honey

<u>Directions:</u>

1. Melt the honey and beeswax in a double boiler on low heat.

2. Remove from heat and add the almond oil then leave to cool slightly.

3. Add the lavender and vanilla oil drops.

4. Pour the mixture carefully into the prepared tins and leave to harden.

5. Rub perfume onto pulse points of skin –neck, forearm and back of knees.

Citrus Lavender Solid Perfume

<u>Ingredients</u>

12 drops sweet orange essential oil

12 drops lemon essential oil

12 drops lavender essential oil

12 drops bergamot essential oil

2 tsp beeswax

2 tsp carrier oil – jojoba or sweet almond oil

Directions:

1. Blend the Essential Oils in a cup

 2. In another cup, add two teaspoons of almond or jojoba oil.

3. Melt the Beeswax in a pot.

4. Add the Carrier Oil, stir until combined.

5. Remove from heat and add essential oils quickly, stirring until just combined.

6. Pour into container, cover and leave to set for about 10 minutes. Enjoy!

Tangerine -Patchouli Solid Perfume

For half-ounce pot of solid perfume

Ingredients

40 drops Tangerine Essential Oil

50 drops Patchouli Essential Oil

5 grams Beeswax

15 ml Jojoba Oil

Directions:

1. In a small shot glass, measure out the jojoba oil.

2. Add essential oils and blend well.

3. Measure out the beeswax. Place it in a small glass and heat it in a water bath until it is melted

4. Remove from the heat but keep the melted beeswax container in the hot water.

5. Pour the essential oil mixture into the melted beeswax.

6. Pour the melted perfume quickly and carefully into a container and leave to harden for about 30 minutes.

7. Label and enjoy.

Sweet Blend Perfume

Ingredients

30 drops Sweet Orange Essential Oil

30 drops Patchouli Essential Oil

30 drops Ylang Ylang Essential Oil

5 grams Beeswax

15 ml Jojoba Oil

Directions:

1. In a small shot glass, measure out the jojoba oil.

2. Add essential oils and blend well.

3. Measure out the beeswax. Place it in a small glass and heat it in a water bath until it is melted

4. Remove from the heat but keep the melted beeswax container in the hot water.

5. Pour the essential oil mixture into the melted beeswax.

6. Pour the melted perfume quickly and carefully into a container and leave to harden for about 30 minutes.

7. Label and enjoy.

Timeout Blend

<u>Ingredients</u>

40 drops lavender Essential Oil

50 drops geranium Essential Oil

5 grams Beeswax

15 ml Jojoba Oil

<u>Directions:</u>

1. in a small shot glass, measure out the jojoba oil.

2. Add essential oils and blend well.

3. Measure out the beeswax. Place it in a small glass and heat it in a water bath until it is melted

4. Remove from the heat but keep the melted beeswax container in the hot water.

5. Pour the essential oil mixture into the melted beeswax.

6. Pour the melted perfume quickly and carefully into a container and leave to harden for about 30 minutes.

7. Label and enjoy.

Woody-Fruity Perfume

Ingredients

30 drops Sandalwood Essential Oil

30 drops Rosewood Essential Oil

30 drops Grapefruit Essential Oil

5 grams Beeswax

15 ml Jojoba Oil

Directions:

1. in a small shot glass, measure out the grapeseed oil or jojoba oil.

2. Add essential oils and blend well.

3. Measure out the beeswax. Place it in a small glass and heat it in a water bath until it is melted

4. Remove from the heat but keep the melted beeswax container in the hot water.

5. Pour the essential oil mixture into the melted beeswax.

6. Pour the melted perfume quickly and carefully into a container and leave to harden for about 30 minutes.

7. Label and enjoy.

HOMEMADE COLOGNE

Citrus Cologne

A revitalizing and stimulating aroma made from fresh citrus.

<u>Ingredients</u>

1 fresh Grapefruit peel, zest only

1 fresh Lemon peel, zest only

Basil, Chamomile, Lavender or Peppermint essential oils

8 oz Vodka

<u>Directions</u>

1. In a glass mason jar, combine the grapefruit and lemon peel zest.

2. Add the vodka until it rises above the peel zest by 1-2 inches.

3. Cap it tightly and shake 2-3 times daily.

4. Leave for 2 to 6 weeks then strain the citrus peels out and pour cologne into a glass bottle.

5. Add 2 drops essential oil per 1 tablespoon of finished cologne.

6. If you want stronger cologne, add more essential oil.

Blooming Floral Cologne

Made with very fresh blossoms, this relaxing cologne helps to ease anxiety, exhaustion, irritability and insomnia.

<u>Ingredients</u>

Rose Petals, fresh or dried

Chamomile flowers, fresh or dried

Lavender flowers, fresh or dried

Vodka

<u>Directions</u>

1. In a glass mason jar, mix together all the ingredients

2. Add the vodka until it rises above the flowers by 1-2 inches.

3. Cap it tightly and shake 2-3 times daily.

4. Leave for 2 to 6 weeks then strain the flowers out.

5. Pour the cologne into a glass bottle

Spicy Orange Cologne

Spicy and exotic, this blend will alleviate mental fatigue, stress, lifts spirits and invigorate senses.

<u>Ingredients</u>

25 organic whole Cardamom Pods

1 organic Cinnamon Stick

1 organic Vanilla Bean, cut into pieces

15 organic Cloves

1 fresh Orange peel, zest only

8 oz Vodka

Directions

1. Use a mortar and pestle to crush the spices.

2. Add the crushed spices to the orange peel zest, vanilla bean pieces and vodka. Combine thoroughly in a mason jar, preferably glass.

3. Cap it tightly and shake 2-3 times daily.

4. Leave for 2 to 6 weeks then strain. Pour the infused liquid into a bottle.

5. If you want stronger cologne, add more spices.

Alpha Male Cologne

Ingredients

15 drops Mandarin or Bergamot

5 drops Bay Laurel

2.5 oz. High Proof Vodka

1 oz. Distilled Water

15 drops Patchouli

3 drops Black Pepper or Ginger

2-3 drops Vetiver or 5 drops Oakmoss Absolute

1-2 drops of Neroli (optional)

Directions:

1. Combine water and alcohol and add to a 4 oz. glass bottle with a sprayer top. Add the oils, shaking well.

2. Let it rest for 5-7days, shaking the bottle twice a day for the oils to blend.

3. Shake the cologne thoroughly before each use. First test it by applying it to a small area in your forearm before fully using.

Rich Spicy Cologne

Ingredients

1 fluid ounce vodka

3 fluid ounces water

8 drops bay essential oil

11 drops bergamot essential oil

2 drops neroli essential oil

3 drops vetiver essential oil

Directions

1. Mix the alcohol, essential oils and water in a glass bottle.

2. Allow the mixture to sit for 2-6 weeks. Shake to mix occasionally.

3. Wear and enjoy.

Lemony Eau De Cologne

<u>Ingredients</u>

10 drops lime oil

3 drops lemongrass oil

10 drops lavender oil

3 ½ fl oz. organic vodka or orrisroot perfume base

<u>Directions</u>

1. Mix all the ingredients together. Let it stand for 48 hours

2. Drip mixture through filter paper then store and tightly seal in a bottle.

3. Alternatively, dilute scent by adding about 50% distilled water to mixture.

Fresh Masculine Cologne

<u>Ingredients</u>

14 drops Petitgrain essential oil

16 drops Bergamot essential oil

8 drops Lemon essential oil

8 drops Orange essential oil

5 drops Neroli essential oil

7 drops Lavender essential oil

10 ml Orange Flower Water

230 ml Vodka or Ethanol Alcohol

Directions

1. Pour the alcohol into a mixing jar.

2. Gently add the essential oils and mix thoroughly.

3. Pour into a dark glass container, seal and set aside for 4 days.

4. Add the orange flower water, cap it and keep from direct sunlight for 2 weeks, shaking lightly daily.

5. Apply Cologne to pulse points where skin is warmest.

Ultra-Rich Eau De Cologne

Ingredients

1.5 ml lemon essential oil

1.5 ml bergamot essential oil

10 drops neroli essential oil

5 drops rosemary essential oil

35 drops orange essential oil

3 1/2 fl oz (100ml) orrisroot perfume base or organic vodka

Directions

1. Mix all the ingredients together. Let it stand for 48 hours

2. Drip mixture through filter paper then store and tightly seal in a bottle.

3. Alternatively, dilute scent by adding about 50% distilled water to mixture.

Homemade Oil Aftershave

While this is not cologne, it is long-lasting and smells great.

<u>Ingredients</u>

5 drops Coriander essential oil

6 drops Bergamot essential oil

1 drop Cedarwood essential oil

3 drops Sandalwood essential oil

4 drops Neroli essential oil

10 ml Jojoba Oil

<u>Directions</u>

1. Pour the jojoba oil in a mixing container.

2. Carefully add the essential oils to it one by one. Mix well.

3. Pour the mixture into small glass container, seal and leave for1 a week.

After-Shave Cologne

Refreshing Alcohol-Free Cologne

<u>Ingredients</u>

2 cups of Witch Hazel Extract

½ oz Vegetable Glycerine

2 oz Rosewater

2 oz Aloe Vera Gel

10 drops Essential Oil of Choice (e.g. sandalwood, lavender, bergamot and peppermint)

Directions

1. Add all ingredients (except the essential oil) to a container and mix thoroughly to combine.

2. Add the essential oil to it and mix well.

3. Re-cap the glass container and shake gently to it.

4. After shaving, pour amount of cologne into your hands and apply gently to face.

5. Avoid the delicate areas of the eye. It may also be used on the pulse points.

PERFUME SPRAYS

Dreamy Perfume Spray

<u>Ingredients</u>

5 drops sandalwood oil

8 drops neroli oil

5 drops mandarin oil

5 drops jasmine oil

1/4 cup distilled water

1/4 cup vodka

<u>Directions</u>

1. Pour all the ingredients into a dark-colored spray bottle. Shake vigorously to mix.

2. Let it stand for 12-18 hours before using.

3. Keep in a cool, dry place.

Blissful Perfume Spray

<u>Ingredients</u>

8 drops freesia essential oil

8 drops vanilla essential oil

1/4 cup distilled water

1/4 cup vodka

5 drops musk oil

<u>Directions</u>

1. Pour all the ingredients into a dark-colored spray bottle. Shake vigorously to mix.

2. Let it stand for 12-18 hours before using.

3. Keep in a cool, dry place.

Fiery Perfume Spray

<u>Ingredients</u>

1/4 cup distilled water

1/4 cup vodka

7 drops amber essential oil

5 drops rosewood essential oil

7 drops myrrh essential oil

5 drops cedar essential oil

<u>Directions</u>

1. Pour all the ingredients into a dark-colored spray bottle. Shake vigorously to mix.

2. Let it stand for 12-18 hours before using.

3. Keep in a cool, dry place.

AROMATHERAPY PERFUMES

Aromatherapy perfumes enhance the mood of the wearer. Depending on the blend, it brings about good mood, drives bad ones away, provides a little energy and calms the mind and body. It may also make the wearer feel feminine, confident, glamorous or exotic.

Below are a few recipes to try:

Aromatherapy Calming Perfume Recipes

1

Ingredients

4 drops Jasmine essential oil

2 drops Lemon essential oil

1 drop Patchouli essential oil

2

Ingredients

2 drops Clary Sage essential oil

4 drops Cedar wood essential oil

2 drops of Mandarin essential oil

1 drop of Grapefruit essential oil

<u>3</u>

<u>Ingredients</u>

3 drops of lavender essential oil

2 drops of Spearmint essential oil

3 drops of Neroli essential oil

<u>Directions</u>

1. Pour all the ingredients into a dark-colored bottle. Shake vigorously to mix.

2. Let it stand for 12-18 hours before using.

3. Keep in a cool, dry place.

Energizing Aromatherapy Perfume

<u>Ingredients</u>

2 drops Grapefruit essential oil

2 drops Patchouli essential oil

2 drops of Ylang-Ylang essential oil

3 drops Vetivert essential oil

1 drop Rose essential oil

<u>Directions</u>

1. Pour all the ingredients into a dark-colored bottle. Shake vigorously to mix.

2. Let it stand for 12-18 hours before using.

3. Keep in a cool, dry place

Tranquilizing Aromatherapy Perfumes

Ingredients

4 drops Lavender essential oil

2 drops Bergamot essential oil

3 drops Chamomile essential oil

2 drops Marjoram essential oil

Directions

1. Pour all the ingredients into a dark-colored bottle. Shake vigorously to mix.

2. Let it stand for 12-18 hours before using.

3. Keep in a cool, dry place

Relaxing Aromatherapy Perfumes

Ingredients

3 drops Jasmine essential oil

4 drops of Orange essential oil

3 drops of Neroli essential oil

OR

2 drops Rose essential oil

3 drops Patchouli essential oil

4 drops Rosewood essential oil

1 drop Clary Sage essential oil

Directions

1. Pour all the ingredients into a dark-colored bottle. Shake vigorously to mix.

2. Let it stand for 12-18 hours before using.

3. Keep in a cool, dry place

SCENTED WATERS

Scented waters are another great way to perfume the body. It can be splashed on after a shower or bath, put in a diffuser bottle and sprayed on the body. What's more, it is simple to make. Here are few recipes to get you started.

Orange Water

<u>Ingredients</u>

1/2 cup orange peel chopped into pieces

1/2 cup vodka

3 cups distilled water

<u>Directions</u>

1. Place the vodka and orange peel in a glass measuring cup. Let it sit for 1day.

2. Use a wooden spoon to mash and then add the distilled water.

3. Let it sit for 1 week but mash and mix it once in a day.

4. Pass the water through a strainer. Pour into a bottle.

5. Use the scented water to perfume your body.

Lemon Water

<u>Ingredients</u>

1/2 cup lemon peel, chopped into pieces

1/2 cup vodka

3 cups distilled water

<u>Directions</u>

1. Place the vodka and orange peel in a glass measuring cup. Let it sit for 1day.

2. Use a wooden spoon to mash and then add the distilled water.

3. Let it sit for 1 week but mash and mix it once in a day.

4. Pass the water through a strainer. Pour into a bottle.

5. Use the scented water to perfume your body.

Rose Water

<u>Ingredients</u>

1/2 cup fresh rose petals

1/2 cup vodka

3 cups distilled water

<u>Directions</u>

1. Place the vodka and rose petals in a glass measuring cup. Let it sit for 1day.

2. Use a wooden spoon to mash and then add the distilled water.

3. Let it sit for 1 week but mash and mix it once in a day.

4. Pass the water through a strainer. Pour into a bottle.

5. Use the scented water to perfume your body.

Lavender Water

<u>Ingredients</u>

1/2 cup fresh lavender flowers

1/2 cup vodka

3 cups distilled water

<u>Directions</u>

1. Place the vodka and lavender flowers in a glass measuring cup. Let it sit for 1day.

2. Use a wooden spoon to mash and then add the distilled water.

3. Let it sit for 1 week but mash and mix it once in a day.

4. Pass the water through a strainer. Pour into a bottle.

5. Use the scented water to perfume your body.

Rosemary Water

<u>Ingredients</u>

1/2 cup chopped fresh rosemary

1/2 cup vodka

3 cups distilled water

Directions

1. Place the vodka and fresh rosemary in a glass measuring cup. Let it sit for 1 day.

2. Use a wooden spoon to mash and then add the distilled water.

3. Let it sit for 1 week but mash and mix it once in a day.

4. Pass the water through a strainer. Pour into a bottle.

5. Use the scented water to perfume your body.

Rosemary Lemon Water

Ingredients

1/4 cup chopped fresh rosemary

1/4 cup lemon peel, chopped into pieces

1/2 cup vodka

3 cups distilled water

Directions

1. Place the vodka and fresh rosemary and lemon peel in a glass measuring cup. Let it sit for 1 day.

2. Use a wooden spoon to mash and then add the distilled water.

3. Let it sit for 1 week but mash and mix it once in a day.

4. Pass the water through a strainer. Pour into a bottle.

5. Use the scented water to perfume your body.

Homemade Perfume For Your Dog

Follow this recipe and your dog will definitely smell fresh all through the day. It repels ticks as well.

Ingredients

15 drops cedarwood essential oil

1 tablespoon beeswax

1 tablespoon vitamin E

Water

Directions

1. Put the beeswax in a mixing bowl then add the vitamin E.

2. Add a little water in a pan and place on the stove. Put the mixing bowl in the saucepan. Let the water boil on high heat until the mixture completely melts.

3. Remove saucepan from heat and the mixing bowl as well.

4. Gradually add the essential oil to your mixture, stirring quickly with a straw so it doesn't harden.

5. Pour the mixture into a container. Let it harder for 30 minutes.

6. Rub the perfume on your dog's collar. Your dog will smell great and will be tick-free.